Contents

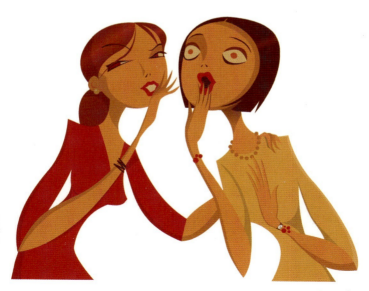

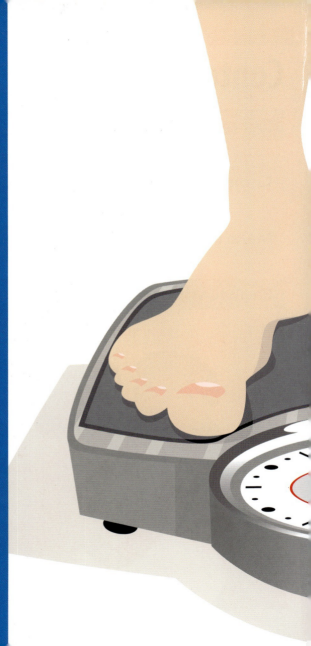

Get motivated, stay motivated

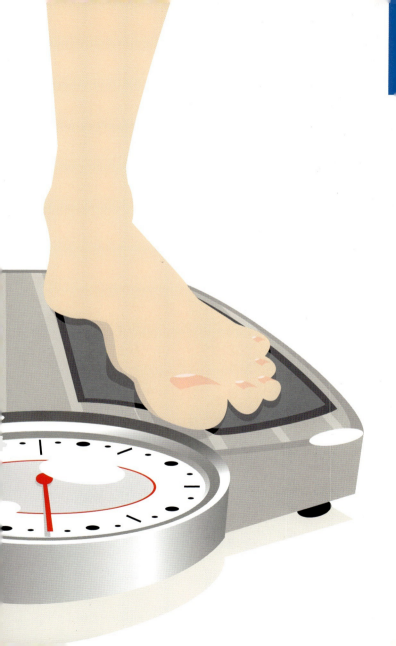

Success breeds success

If you've ever struggled with weight loss (and most of us have at one time or another!) you might get to the stage where you wonder whether it's really possible.

It most certainly is, and one of the best ways of re-affirming it in your own mind is to read the success stories of other slimmers.

Look through the latest issue of Boost! magazine or go online to www.scottishslimmers.com, and be inspired by some amazing achievements.

Learn about obstacles that have been overcome - often against all the odds – and take comfort in the knowledge that these are ordinary folk like you and me. Most didn't get it right all the time, but they are proof that perseverance works.

If they can do it, there is absolutely no reason why you can't also – and what's more, if you have overcome difficulties or have a story that could inspire others, you too could have a fabulous makeover day and find yourself on the pages of Boost!

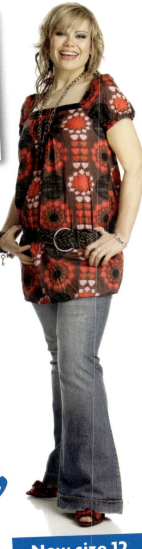

Then size 34

Lisa Milburn

"It's still a shock to see myself looking as glamorous as this! Going to the class and following the Positive Eating Plan was part of my life but I have to confess that my health was no longer my motivation. Health had definitely been replaced by vanity!"

Weight loss:
18 stone

Now size 12

Make a date

We're not terribly in favour of anyone saying they must be at a certain weight by a certain date – things happen, and it can be very de-motivating if after a few weeks you realise that there is no way on earth you can possibly achieve your target.

Scottish Slimmers

2008

SUNDAY	MONDAY	TUESDAY	WEDNESDAY	THURSDAY	FRIDAY	SATURDAY
1	2	3	4	5	6	7
8	9	10	11	12	13	14
15	16	17	18	19	20	21
22	23	24	25 TODAY	26	27	28
29	30	31	1	2	3	4

But, many slimmers do find it helpful to have a special date or occasion in mind, such as a wedding, birthday, holiday or Christmas, by which time they want to have lost some weight.

Such dates are not reasons for wanting to lose weight permanently, but it's quite a good strategy to get you through a few weeks or months at a time.

Of course, when the occasion has passed, you'll need to think of another suitable date to get you through the next chunk of weight loss!

Do it with a friend

It's a very rare thing indeed if you are the only person in a group who wants to lose weight, so why not suggest to someone that you do it together.

You can share success and encourage each other should you have a disappointment. And sometimes even a little bit of competition might be just what you need to keep you on the straight and narrow!

If you don't feel comfortable doing it with people you know, joining a Scottish Slimmers class is a great way of meeting other like-minded people and you'll almost certainly find a pal who is going through the same difficulties as you.

If you can't get to a class, how about joining an online community (try www.scottishslimmers.com). It's incredible how you only have to mention that you need a little bit of extra encouragement, or have a query or niggle and, before you know it, you get a whole range of reassuring comments and personal advice from those who have been there and are more than willing to share their experience with you and give you their support.

It's a lot more fun when you know you are not alone!

Picture it

If you have a photo of a slimmer you that you would like to return to, why not post it up on your mirror so that each day you get a visual reminder of where you are going.

If you don't have a picture of yourself, you could use an image of someone you would like to look like!

Some people find that putting the photo on the freezer or kitchen cupboard reminds them not to sneak another dollop of ice cream or packet of crisps!

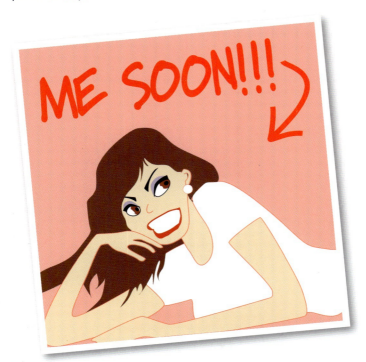

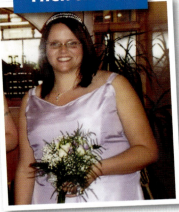

Then size 20

Kirsty Johnstone

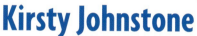

" **Exercise has really helped me - I even get loads of exercise on a night out because I'm never off the dance floor! More Dancing, less dinner.** "

Weight loss:
4 stone 1 lb

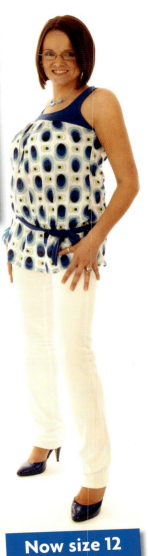

Now size 12

Picture it again – and again

Most of us fight shy of the camera if we are unhappy about our weight but, in these days of digital cameras and cameras on phones, why not pluck up the courage and get someone to take a full-length photo of you every week whilst you are losing weight.

From week to week there won't be much difference, but after a few weeks it's fun to compare with pictures from the first week or two.

You won't want to print off all the photos, but what a fantastic record you'll have of your journey if, for example, you wanted to enter our Slimmer of the Year competition.

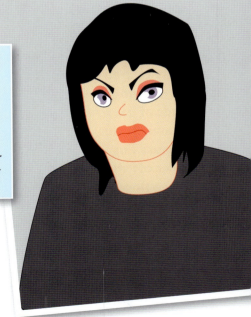

How long is a piece of string?

Take a piece of string, put it around your waist and cut to size.

Remember that your weight on the scales is not the only indicator of your success. If ever you are disappointed with your weight loss, take out your piece of string, put it around your waist and either feel the gap, or note how much extra string you now have.

You don't even have to put a number on it – you just know you are making good progress.

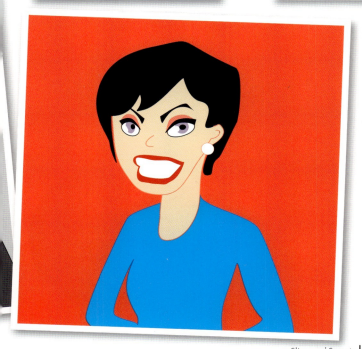

The last straw

Do you remember what it was that made you really want to lose weight this time?

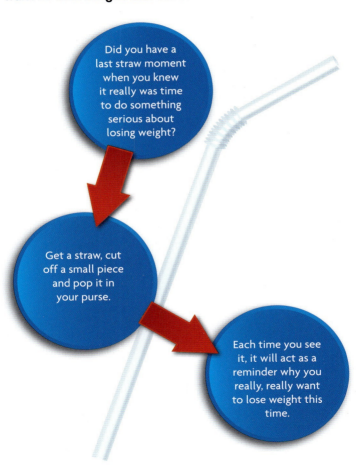

Did you have a last straw moment when you knew it really was time to do something serious about losing weight?

Get a straw, cut off a small piece and pop it in your purse.

Each time you see it, it will act as a reminder why you really, really want to lose weight this time.

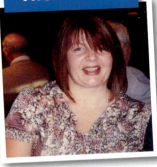

Then size 22

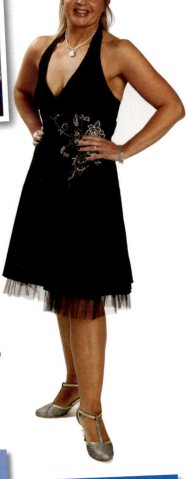

Fiona Smith

" **Running is my slimming secret – it gives me some time to myself and I feel so good afterwards.** "

Weight loss: 2 stone 11 lbs

Now size 12

See how far you've come

If you've been losing weight for several weeks or months – and still have a way to go, it can seem that there's no light at the end of the tunnel.

This is the time to step back and think about how far you have come rather than how far you still have to go.

In addition to the amount of weight you've lost, have you made any positive changes to your habits or lifestyle that you think you will live with permanently? If you have, that's a real achievement.

Also remember that your weight loss is much bigger than you think. If you hadn't done anything about your weight over the past few weeks or months, chances are you would now weigh a lot more than you did when you started.

So your efforts count not only for the pounds you have lost over the past few weeks, but also for the pounds that you probably would have gained in that time!

Keep fat in the fridge

We're often quite surprised when we hear someone say, "I've only lost a pound".

A pound of fat is a lot of fat!

Keep a pound of fat in the fridge (alright, in this day and age it will probably be a 500g block which is just a fraction more than a pound).

If ever you hear yourself saying "I've only lost a pound", take your pound of fat out of the fridge and place it on your hips or tum and ask yourself if you would rather have it back – or are you glad to see the back of it?

An average loss of:

½ lb a week is 26 lb or nearly 2 stones in a year

1 lb a week is 52 lb or 3 st 10 lb in a year

1½ lb a week is 78 lb or 5 st 8 lb in a year

2 lb a week is 104 lb or 7 st 6lb in a year!

A pound of fat is a lot of fat!

Graphic

It can be really inspiring to see a graph of your weekly weight loss with that line going down and down.

You might think, what happens if I have a bad week and the line goes up!

Don't panic, it should simply act as a reminder for you to check that you are keeping up with all your good habits –

Are you keeping to reasonable portion sizes?

Are you eating healthy foods most of the time?

Are you staying within your Check allowance?

Are you trying to be more active?

If you are letting things slip, that could be why the line has gone up – and if you nip it in the bud, the line will soon take a downward turn.

If you haven't let things slip, and continue to put in the same amount of effort as you have been, you can rest assured it will only be a blip, and that line will go down again.

It doesn't necessarily have to be a dead straight line to prove it's working – just a general trend in a downward direction.

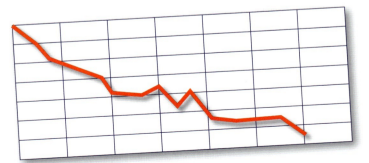

Take on a challenge

Many people find that taking on the challenge of a sponsored walk or run is just the motivation they need to go the extra mile – both figuratively and literally!

Preparing for the event (training, if you like) often means you make a regular commitment to some additional exercise which will make you fitter and help boost your weight loss.

If you're not sure where to begin, or how to get involved, try clicking on one of the following:

www.jogscotland.org.uk

www.raceforlife.org

www.walkthewalk.org

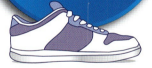

Show 'em!

There are many good reasons for losing weight associated with your health and improving your life, but if these are not enough to inspire you, you might get off the starting blocks, and hopefully keep going to the finishing line, if now and again you remind yourself of someone to whom you would really like to prove that you can do it!

Your boss, your ex, your sister, your brother, your "friend", that shop assistant who gave you a funny look?

Don't let their comments or attitude knock your confidence. If you struggle with your weight it's easy to forget that you're really rather good at other things.

Think about all the things you do well — coping with a difficult or stressful job, making time for the children, entertaining your friends, playing a sport or musical instrument, managing a household budget, fantastic at putting on eye make-up or a whiz with hair, knowing how to put other people at ease, fixing things.

We bet there are loads of things, big and small, that you do really well and which you never give yourself credit for. Think about those things — and better still, write a list of them.

If you can do all those things, there's no reason why you can't lose weight!

So, go show 'em!

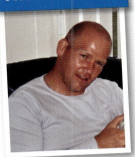

Then waist 40

Paul Robinson

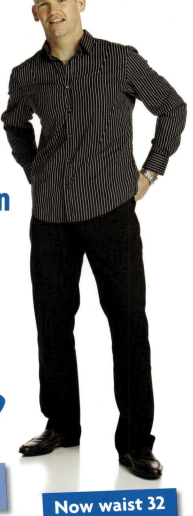

" I swapped lager for a cup of coffee and fruit when I get home – knowing I would have a filling and delicious home-cooked meal later on. "

Weight loss:
4 stone

Now waist 32

If it didn't fit yesterday...
... it might fit today!

Do you have something in your wardrobe that you used to love wearing and felt really good in, but unfortunately you just can't get into now?

As the pounds come off, keep trying it on.

It's really motivating when you can do up another button or the zip goes up a bit further.

Also remember that as you lose weight and your clothes become looser and looser, they might not be doing you justice. You don't have to wait until you reach Target Weight before buying something new! Even the odd item from a charity shop or supermarket in a size smaller can lift your spirits and boost your morale no end. Try it!

Measure up

Take your measurements at least once a month and make a note of them. It will act as reassurance that your weight loss plan is working — even if the scales are unkind to you sometimes.

Remember that to reduce health risks, we are advised that women should keep their waist measurement below 32 inches (80 cm) and men should keep their waist below 37 inches (94 cm).

Another different way of monitoring your progress is to use body fat monitor scales, but if you use these, do be prepared for regular fluctuations up or down by a percentage or two because the reading is dependent on the amount of fluid in your body at any given time. You should always weigh at the same time of day under the same conditions (e.g. first thing in the morning after having gone to the loo). Note your progress, say, once every couple of weeks or once a month rather than every day or week.

The following are based on National Institutes of Health/World Health Organisation guidelines:

Age	Under Fat	Healthy	Over Fat	Obese
Women				
20 – 39	less than 21%	21% - 33%	33% - 39%	over 39%
40 – 59	less than 23%	23% - 34%	34% - 40%	over 40%
60 – 79	less than 24%	24% - 36%	36% - 42%	over 42%
Men				
20 – 39	less than 8%	8% - 20%	20% - 25%	over 25%
40 – 59	less than 11%	11% - 22%	22% - 28%	over 28%
60 – 79	less than 13%	13% - 25%	25% - 30%	over 30%

Spot the difference

As you lose weight, it's not only the number on the scales that changes. Look out for other signs of success:

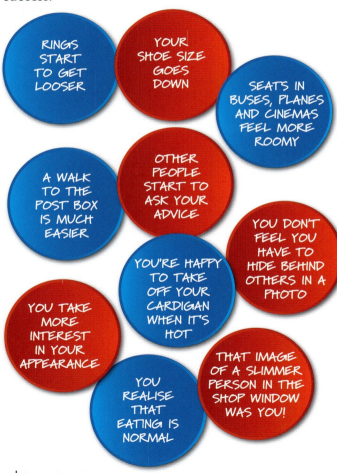

RINGS START TO GET LOOSER

YOUR SHOE SIZE GOES DOWN

SEATS IN BUSES, PLANES AND CINEMAS FEEL MORE ROOMY

A WALK TO THE POST BOX IS MUCH EASIER

OTHER PEOPLE START TO ASK YOUR ADVICE

YOU DON'T FEEL YOU HAVE TO HIDE BEHIND OTHERS IN A PHOTO

YOU'RE HAPPY TO TAKE OFF YOUR CARDIGAN WHEN IT'S HOT

YOU TAKE MORE INTEREST IN YOUR APPEARANCE

THAT IMAGE OF A SLIMMER PERSON IN THE SHOP WINDOW WAS YOU!

YOU REALISE THAT EATING IS NORMAL

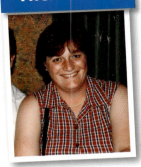

Then size 18

Karen Roger

" I plan all my meals and cook myself - rather than go for a quick but bland ready meal Do it so that it became an enjoyable part of your day! "

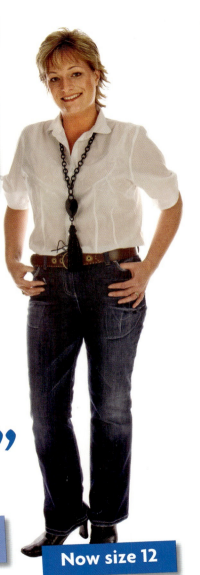

Now size 12

Weight loss:
5 stone

With compliments

When we're overweight we often feel insignificant or have low self-esteem. Remember that nobody else is perfect either!

We tend to think that everything will be different once we have lost weight. Well, there certainly will be many differences, but don't underestimate your value now. Whilst losing weight often gives you the confidence to try out new things, it is equally true that having self-confidence is a great asset when it comes to weight loss.

Instead of always being on the defensive, take note of when people pay you compliments – it means they value you.

It's a compliment when someone says, "You look nice today".

It's a compliment when someone wants your opinion about something.

It's a compliment when someone says, "I couldn't have done it without you".

It's a compliment when someone says, "How did you do that?"

It's a compliment when people say, "We need you".

You deserve it!

Frankly, few things in life give so many people so much pleasure as seeing their weight on the scales go down!

But losing weight takes effort and it's only right that your efforts should be rewarded.

Some people tell us that their partners promise them something like a holiday or a weekend away or some other special treat to look forward to when they reach Target Weight. Lucky them!

But you don't have to wait until you reach Target Weight.

Even if you have just a stone or so to lose, plan to buy yourself a little treat for every four or five pounds you lose. It's good if you think about your treats in advance so you can enjoy the anticipation.

If you have several stones to lose, how about something for every half stone loss? You could increase the value of each item along the way so you end up with something you really, really want when you reach Target Weight.

Or, another popular incentive is to squirrel away a pound (or five!) for every 1lb weight loss – because you're sure to want to go on a spending spree for a few new outfits to flatter your Target Weight figure.

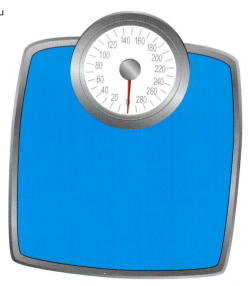

Happy to be healthy

If you feel well it's easy to forget the impact that being overweight can have on your health.

You may feel fine now, but if your weight increases you put your health at risk in many ways. It's better to take action now, before it becomes an issue.

Being overweight increases the health risks associated with:

✔ HIGH BLOOD PRESSURE

✔ STROKE

✔ HIGH CHOLESTEROL

✔ HEART DISEASE

✔ DIABETES

✔ ARTHRITIS

✔ COMPLICATIONS IN PREGNANCY

More recently the effects of being overweight on various types of cancer are becoming clearer especially in respect of cancer of the bowel, breast cancer in post-menopausal women, cancer of the oesophagus (food pipe), kidney and womb. There also appear to be links with overweight and cancer of the pancreas, gallbladder, prostate, thyroid, ovaries and liver.

You owe it to yourself to look after your health.

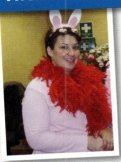

Then size 18

Jayne Booth

" I never used to exercise, but to help my weight loss I started to walk and now I love it -- the fresh air and time to myself is great. "

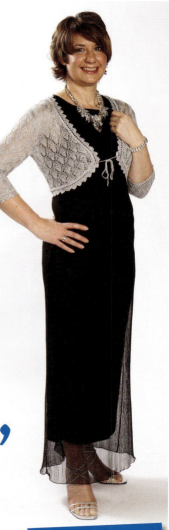

**Weight loss:
3 stone 5 lbs**

Now size 12

Fat suits

You may have seen celebs on telly donning fat suits laden with weights equal to the amount of weight they have lost. Walking around in them for a little while soon makes them appreciate the benefits of losing surplus pounds.

You can have a similar experience simply by loading up a couple of shopping bags either with potatoes or canned foods or stones equivalent to the pounds you've shed.

Try walking around with them for 10-15 minutes, or going up and down the stairs a few times. You'll find it hard to believe how you managed before.

Losing two or three stones is the equivalent of not having to permanently carry a toddler around with you all day!

Naughty knickers!

Do you have a dream of wearing a particular item of clothing?

We were once inspired by a granny who told us she had always wanted to wear a little pair of knickers with tie strings at the sides – and she told us that having reached Target Weight, the first thing she did was go out and buy herself a pair!

Maybe you dream about looking fantastic in a pair of jeans, or looking good in a swimsuit, or want to make sure you look like a princess on your wedding day.

Keep thinking about it, and if you want it enough – you'll get it!

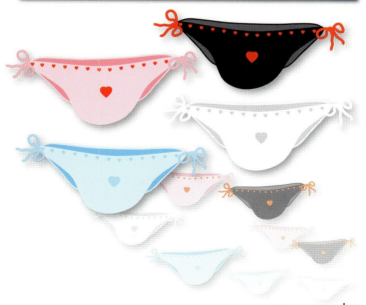

Coping

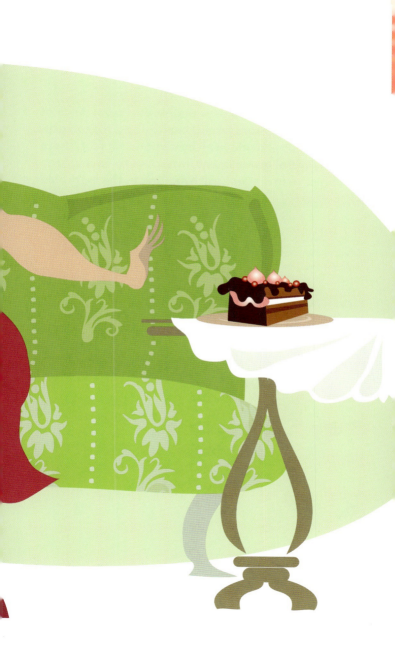

Lunch at work

Many employers these days realise the importance of keeping their workers fit and healthy and try to ensure their canteens provide healthy options. In fact, there are now several government initiatives to encourage employers to invest in healthy eating in the workplace.

Even so, some healthier alternatives may still be higher in Checks than you can afford whilst trying to lose weight. Watch out for:

Salads already dressed with oily vinaigrette.

Portions of sunflower spread that are not low-fat.

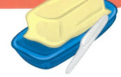

Low-fat yoghurts are not a bad choice, but will have a higher Check value than "diet" or "virtually-fat-free" varieties.

Semi-skimmed milk is better than full-fat milk, but not as low as skimmed milk.

Stir-fries will probably have been cooked with more oil than you would use at home.

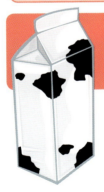

Minced meat in chilli or spaghetti Bolognese may not be as lean as you would choose.

The safest option is to take your own – there are plenty of suggestions in the PEP. It really is just a question of getting organised.

Make sure you have some suitable containers that transport food safely without leaking.

Prepare your lunch the night before to save time in the morning.

Keep a can opener in your office drawer.

Always try to include something starchy (bread, cooked rice or pasta), some protein (lean meat, poultry, tinned fish, hard-boiled eggs, low-fat cheese, beans) and some salad and/or fruit.

A local supermarket is a good place to pop out to for a low-calorie sandwich or salad and some fruit if you've really not had time to prepare anything.

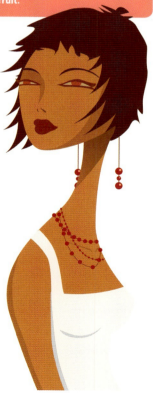

You'll save a lot of money as well as saving Checks – saving a couple of pounds a day for a year is enough for a two-week holiday!

Planes and trains

Most of us don't fly that often, so it's unlikely that any meal eaten on a flight is going to have a serious impact on our long-term weight. And, let's face it, meals are often not that appetising, and portion sizes are generally restricted even if we do eat everything.

Most airlines will cater for special dietary needs if ordered at time of booking, but ordering a vegetarian meal won't necessarily mean a lower-Check meal.

Do take care with alcohol though. That's one way you could bump up the Checks. Flying is dehydrating and so is alcohol, so it's really not a good combination anyway. Drinking plenty of water, however, is a good idea. So, if restrictions on liquids are still in force, you'll need to buy some, or another sugar-free drink, after passport control to take on board with you.

If you are taking a domestic flight on a no-frills airline at a time when you need to eat, you can often pick up a "meal deal" after passport control at Boots – but ensure you choose from their Shapers range! This will save you loads of Checks compared with the usual array of baguettes, stuffed croissants, pizza slices or burgers normally on offer at other outlets.

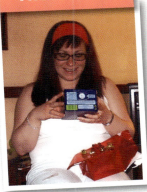

Then size 14

Julie Hamill

" I bought as many recipes books as I could – and I have enjoyed trying all sorts of new meals which has meant that I have never been bored and never been hungry. "

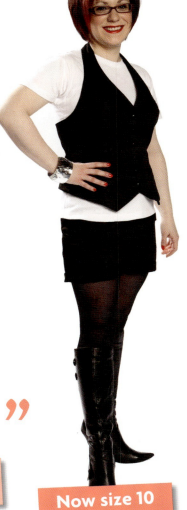

Weight loss:
2 stone 6 lbs

Now size 10

Hostess with the mostest

When we're the hostess, we often feel that the more we lavish on our guests, the more they will appreciate our efforts. In this day and age, when so many of us are trying to watch our waistlines, or are at least aiming to take a few steps in the right direction, our guests are more likely to appreciate food that enables them to stay on track.

If you are looking to please:

Provide light wines that can be spritzed with diet mixers or soda.

Vegetable soups or seafood salads make light starters – allow guests to add their own dressings. Offer low-fat or olive oil spreads instead of butter to go with any bread or toast.

Great quality fish, poultry or lean meat cooked simply without the addition of a rich creamy sauce are usually appreciated. Sauces could be tomato-based or made from stock and a little wine. Garlic and fresh herbs will add flavour.

New potatoes or home-made wedges are lighter than roast or creamy mash. Or if mash is what suits, make with skimmed milk and try adding chopped spring onion, or finely chopped herbs, or grated lemon zest.

Provide lots of steamed veg, or oven-roasted veg cooked with a few sprays of oil rather than drizzling oil all over.

If you feel you must offer dessert make it light and fruity, or at least offer fresh fruit or fruit salad as an alternative. Low-fat Greek yoghurt, or fromage frais, or a little half-fat crème fraîche make good toppings.

Don't be scared to offer meals from the Positive Eating Plan! If, however, you are going to be cooking for several guests, and will need to quadruple quantities or more, we suggest you have a practice run beforehand, as the amount of liquid needed for a recipe and length of cooking time may vary from those given for single-serving meals. (You'll probably be able to freeze leftover portions for an easy meal for another time.)

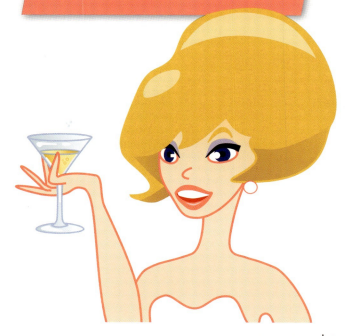

Saving Checks

Ask any Scottish Slimmer and they will probably tell you that saving Checks is one of the best strategies available to anyone with a busy social life!

It's not wise to try and cut back too severely on any one day in order to save lots and lots of Checks. The best way is to try and save about 3-5 Checks a day for 4 or 5 days prior to a social event where you know you would like to eat a little more than usual.

This should give you around 15-20 saved Checks to spend. If you add these to your normal daily allowance of Checks on the day of the event, and if you choose carefully for your other meals on that day, and make full use of your Every Day Bonus foods, you should easily be able to afford a couple of drinks and perhaps a dessert or starter in addition to a nice main course for a special meal out.

A bowl or two of soup made with No-Check veggies before heading out can take the edge off your appetite and make it easier to stick with your good intentions.

It's a good idea to try and plan in advance how you intend to spend your saved Checks. That way you can anticipate the enjoyment and knowing the boundaries will also make it less likely you will overindulge.

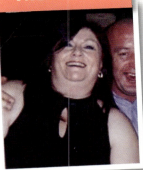

Paula Stalker

" I love my food which is why I love the PEPplus plan – my top tip is 'Enjoy everything you eat'. "

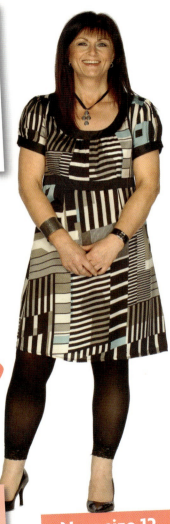

Weight loss:
7 stone 11 lbs

Now size 12

Allow yourself some leeway

Sometimes you can find yourself in a situation where you know you will be eating more Checks than you should but have not had time to save any Checks in advance.

THE WORST THING YOU CAN DO IS SIMPLY DECIDE THAT YOU ARE GOING TO OVER-EAT ANYWAY, SO YOU MIGHT AS WELL DO IT BIG TIME!

A simple solution is to allow yourself an extra 15-20 Checks to cope with the situation.

The object of the exercise is to keep things within reasonable bounds.

TRY AND SPEND THE EXTRA CHECKS WISELY, AND IF YOU ARE UNSURE ABOUT THE CHECK VALUE OF THE FOOD YOU ARE EATING, GUESS A REASONABLE VALUE.

If, however, you do this on a regular basis, your weight loss will slow down and it means that you are not really taking your normal lifestyle into account and planning in advance.

BUT AS AN OCCASIONAL COPING MECHANISM, AN EXTRA 15-20 CHECKS IN A WEEK WILL ONLY SLOW DOWN YOUR REAL, LONG-TERM WEIGHT LOSS BY ABOUT 2-3 OUNCES.

Have it on credit

This is a little secret that some slimmers find helpful – but it's not for everyone.

For whatever reason, you know that you've had a few too many Checks on one day.

You can simply to forget it and get right back on track with your usual plan. Nobody is perfect, and drawing a line under it and getting on with life is a far better way than saying "I was bad, so I might as well be awful!"

If you don't want to lose ground, you could also try to make up for some, if not all, of your over-spend.

If you regularly keep a note of how you spend your Checks, work out roughly how many Checks too many you've had. Then, write them in, spread out over the next few days.

For example, let's say on Monday you had 3 packets of crisps instead of the 1 packet you intended. You could write in 1 packet of crisps on Tuesday and another on Wednesday. It will mean you have a few less Checks to spend on those days, but you will still be able to keep to your weekly total Checks.

In practice, you would be saving Checks in arrears instead of advance – or, if you like, having it on credit.

Pub grub

Pubs can be a bit of a minefield when trying to lose weight! Not only do you need to keep tabs on the amount of alcohol you drink but, traditionally, their menus include a lot of very hearty stuff, often with quite generous portions.

But times are changing and it is often possible to find something lighter.

If there is a salad bar, fill your bowl mostly with fresh salad vegetables, then add a tablespoon or two of your favourite oil or mayonnaise-dressed salad, if you really must, but note that each heaped tablespoon is likely to cost you in the region of 3 Checks.

Soups are often a good choice for a starter, provided they are not "cream of". A roll and a pat of butter will cost 8 or 9 Checks, so think carefully before you indulge. Prawn and avocado cocktails, nachos, anything breaded and deep-fried such as mushrooms or camembert, pasta starters and almost any type of pâté will be some of the highest Check items on the starter menu.

Salmon, any fish (no batter), poultry or game birds with skin removed or a lean grilled steak are the best choices for a main course. Be cautious about quiches and tarts, or vegetarian risottos that could have a lot of butter and cheese added.

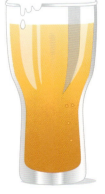

Berries, fresh fruit salad or sorbets will be the safest choices for dessert. Or, if you have a fellow slimmer with you, you could perhaps share something a little more indulgent.

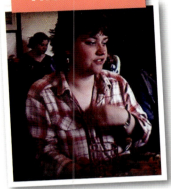

Then size 16

Ali Smith

❝ **Go to class every week – and don't be too hard on yourself.** ❞

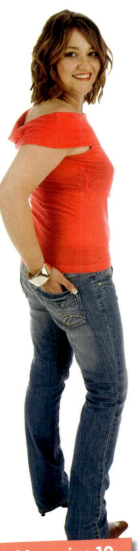

Weight loss:
3 stone

Now size 10

Choosing Chinese

The secret of picking your way through a Chinese menu is firstly to avoid anything that is battered and deep-fried such as sweet & sour chicken or pork balls or crispy shredded beef. Other deep-fried items will also bump up the Checks – spring rolls or pancake rolls, sesame prawn toast or crispy seaweed.

Anything in sweet & sour sauce is likely to be low-fat, but often contains a lot of sugar which can put up the Checks.

The best choices are usually based on chicken, prawns, tofu or beef that have been stir-fried with various vegetables. They will contain at least 1 tablespoon of oil per serving, but this is often peanut oil, which is fairly high in good monounsaturates, like olive oil, but not at all suitable if you have a nut allergy.

Chinese food is also not a good choice if you have been advised to follow a low-sodium diet, or have high blood pressure, as soy sauce is really high in salt. 1 tablespoon of soy sauce contains almost half the recommended daily maximum for salt.

The best choice for rice is, obviously, plain boiled, but a takeaway portion of egg fried rice (roughly 250-300g) is likely to be only about 4 Checks more than the equivalent amount of boiled rice and may be worth it for the extra satisfaction.

And, if you are really intent on keeping to your weight loss plan, don't even start on the prawn crackers – or be prepared to count half a Check for each one!

Into Indian

Indian food can be very high in Checks because it is often cooked with lots of oil, and may also contain coconut milk (very high in saturated fat) or have ghee (clarified butter, also high in saturated fat) added at the end. Portion sizes are usually quite substantial too!

When ordering, consider whether or not you really need a starter. If you must, a poppadum with a teaspoon of pickles, chutney or raita is a reasonable choice, or go for something dry such as a starter portion of chicken tikka or chicken tandoori (unless you intend to have these for your main course).

When it comes to main courses, go for chicken, prawn or vegetable curries rather than meat, especially lamb which can be very fatty. Korma or butter sauces are likely to be highest in Checks, balti, bhuna, jalfrezi or rogan josh likely to be lowest.

Vegetable side dishes are also usually quite high in Checks being cooked in lots of oil and, if cooked slowly, will have a lot of their vitamin content depleted. If available, it may be a healthier option to finish your meal with some fresh mango or pineapple (and be sure to have an extra portion of veg tomorrow!).

Choose either bread (a medium chapatti at about 5 or 6 Checks is much lower than a naan at 15-20 Checks) or rice – you don't really need both!

Eating out in an Indian restaurant for a social occasion is one thing, but do you really need to call the local takeaway? If you look in your local supermarket, there are so many "healthy" versions of Indian meals that you can keep in the freezer. The advantage is that you can convert calorie information into Checks and be more sure of what you are really eating. And what's more, they can often be microwaved and on your table in less time than it takes the local takeaway to deliver! Definitely worth considering.

Special Diets

Many Scottish Slimmer members have successfully lost weight following not only the Positive Eating Plan but also taking into account their own special dietary needs at the same time.

Here are their tips for success:

FIRST find out from your doctor or dietician which foods you are or are not allowed to eat (you need to know this whether or not you are trying to lose weight).

GO through the PEP and mark the meals you know are suitable for you.

NOTE the meals that you could possibly include if you made one or two simple alterations. In most instances making a substitution, such as swapping ordinary wheat pasta for corn or rice pasta, will make very little difference to the Check value of a meal.

FIND out which special products are available in your local supermarket or health food shop that might be helpful. Most large supermarkets have a "Free From…" section.

CHECK the nutrition information on special products. 1 Check is approximately 25 calories so you can convert calories into Checks by dividing them by 25 – or take the pack into class and ask your Class Manager to help!

GET to know the Check values of everyday basic foods, so you can start to make up your own suitable meals and recipes.

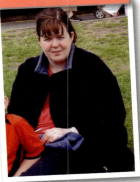

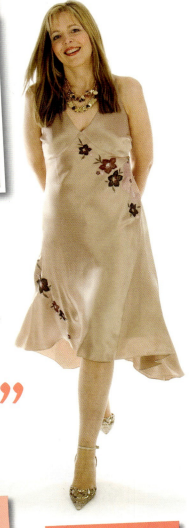

Evelyn Schoppler

" I cooked the same meals for the whole family to make sure I kept to the plan. "

Weight loss:
6 stone 9 lbs

Now size 12

Coping with cravings

A food craving is an intense desire for a particular food rather than food in general. Whilst experts are not really sure what causes cravings, there are some possible theories.

One is that your body tries to make up for nutritional deficiencies by craving a particular food rich in a nutrient in which you are deficient. The theory breaks down somewhat in that popular cravings tend to be for foods such as ice cream, crisps and chocolate which are not very nutrient-dense!

If the craving is for a starchy or sugary food, it is more likely that fluctuating blood sugar levels are to blame. Foods high in sugar and refined starch (generally high GI foods), set off a vicious cycle where blood sugar levels rise rapidly, giving immediate satisfaction, but then drop rapidly leaving you craving more of the same.

To avoid this syndrome, it's a good idea to eat a variety of foods at the same meal. Choose from lower GI carbs such as basmati rice, brown rice, wholemeal, granary or pitta bread, oat-based cereals, pasta, peas and beans. Adding some protein (lean meat, fish, eggs, low-fat dairy, soya products) helps to slow things down even more, as will the fibre in fruits and veg. Good fats such as those found in olive oil or rapeseed oil also slow down stomach emptying, as do acidic foods such as vinegar or lemon juice (ideal for salad dressings). Eating these slow-release foods keeps blood sugar levels more stable.

Following very low-calorie "crash" diets will also cause blood sugar levels to drop rapidly making the desire to eat very intense. If the diet is also very restrictive, forbidding particular foods or groups of food, there is likely to be a strong psychological desire to binge on the forbidden foods.

Cravings are particularly common at times of hormonal change, particularly when women are pre-menstrual, or are pregnant, or sometimes in post-menopausal women. It's not surprising that men don't appear to suffer from cravings as intensely or as frequently as women!

Possibly the best ways of dealing with cravings are:

Eat as healthily as possible at all times, to eliminate possible nutritional deficiencies.

Eat a variety of foods including lower GI carbs. Space food out regularly throughout the day and never crash diet. These strategies will help stabilise blood sugar levels. Eating sufficient good carbs (rather than refined white starchy or sugary carbs) will also help maintain levels of serotonin, a feel-good hormone.

Don't completely deny yourself your favourite foods, as you don't want to start a psychological craving. Equally, avoid using food as a reward, which may be how we become psychologically addicted to a particular food in the first place.

Don't underestimate the value of regular exercise. Done at a moderate pace, exercise releases endorphins, often called happy hormones, which relieve stress and give a feeling of contentment.

If a genuine, very intense craving should arise, it is unlikely you will satisfy it by trying to eat something else. It's probably better to allow yourself a controlled amount of the desired food rather than eating something else and then eating the desired food as well!

If, however, you try to follow the above suggestions on an ongoing basis, you may be able to avoid the cravings happening in the first place.

PMS

There are well over 100 symptoms associated with pre-menstrual syndrome (PMS) but it is not understood why some women only suffer symptoms such as mild irritability whilst others suffer symptoms that affect their life profoundly.

If you are severely affected by symptoms such as migraine, depression, bloating, breast tenderness, crying for no apparent reason or any other symptom that seriously affects your life adversely, you should speak to your GP who may be able to prescribe medication that offers relief, or may advise an over-the-counter supplement such as evening primrose oil or vitamin B6 supplements.

If you find it very difficult to stay within your allowed level of Checks during this time and frequently find yourself eating a lot more than you should, you may find it helpful to consciously allow yourself an extra 5 or 10 Checks a day for your worst few days each month rather than go off the rails completely. This will slow down your weight loss slightly – but nowhere near as much as a week of uncontrolled bingeing!

Symptoms are due to fluctuating levels of hormones in the week (or two) prior to the onset of a period and are real. Due to fluid retention, some women can gain as much as 5-7lb whilst 1-2lb is more usual. It can be quite discouraging to see a gain on the scales at this time, especially if you have tried very hard and have overcome the desire to eat more. Fluid weight gained disappears in the first half of the menstrual period, so it cannot be blamed for cumulative weight gain. Cutting back on salt, salty condiments and seasonings and high salt processed foods will help reduce fluid retention.

On an ongoing basis, eating a healthy diet, including lower GI carbs, and spacing meals evenly throughout the day – as suggested in "Coping with Cravings" – is the best thing you can do personally to help relieve symptoms. Reducing your intake of alcohol and caffeine-containing drinks may also help.

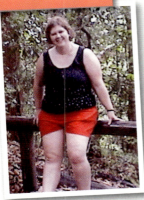

Irene Munro

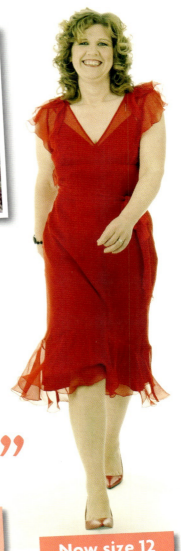

> **I travel a lot which made losing over 5 stone very difficult, so I saved my Checks to cover difficult times when I am flying all over the world for my job.**

Weight loss:
5 stone 3 lbs

Now size 12

Hunger-busting

There's nothing wrong with eating when you're hungry – but the best policy is to try and avoid becoming excessively hungry in the first place!

Don't confuse hunger with appetite. Appetite is when you just fancy eating something, often in response to a trigger such as seeing food, or smelling it or even just talking about it. Real hunger starts when you haven't eaten for a few hours and perhaps your tummy starts to rumble and you start to notice a lack of concentration.

Before eating something, a good question to ask yourself is, "Do I want this – or do I need this?" – and eat it only if you need it!

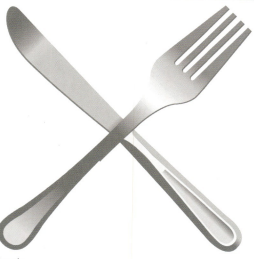

If you skip breakfast, it's an almost dead-cert that you will feel hungry before lunchtime. It's not too much of a problem if you are able to take breakfast with you to have before you start work, or to have mid-morning. But, if you know there will be no opportunity to eat before lunch, you are really setting yourself up for failure if you skip breakfast. Extreme hunger will take over and you will have eaten twice as much as you should before you even realise it.

Another good tip is to get to know at what times of the day you usually feel hungry. If it's outside a normal mealtime, it makes sense to set aside a few Checks for a planned snack. Many people find they have a dip around 4-o'-clock in the afternoon, and many others feel they need a snack before bedtime.

When it comes to hunger-busting meals, as we've previously said, the best choice is a mixture of healthy, wholesome carbs (such as brown or basmati rice, jacket potatoes, pasta, wholegrain breads) and protein foods (such as lean meat, fish, eggs, dairy-foods, peas and beans) that will sustain you for longer by releasing their energy over a longer period of time. Couple these with lots of No-Check vegetables for immediate bulk and satisfaction and you have the perfect hunger-busting combination!

Keep taking the pills!

Many of us try to lose weight to improve our health, so it can be really frustrating if we need to take medication that hinders our effort.

It's worth noting that any one type of drug does not necessarily have the same effect on different people and also that there is often a choice of drugs available to treat the same condition. So, if you feel your medication is making you gain weight, or hindering your weight loss, do speak to your GP who may be able to choose an alternative.

Never stop taking prescribed medication unless advised by your GP.

Is it worth continuing if you feel you are fighting an uphill battle? We feel it is.

Weight gain due to medication is likely to be in the order of a few pounds, but if you also continue to over-eat, you'll add even more weight that you can't blame on the pills, and should you be able to stop taking the medication, you'll have even more surplus weight to deal with.

Try not to be too concerned about the length of time it is taking. More important is to change to a healthier way of eating that you can live with permanently. Weight loss is just the bonus and it doesn't really matter how long it takes to reach Target Weight – because you intend staying there permanently!

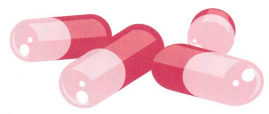

In for the long haul

Losing weight takes time! And, if you wish to lose a lot of weight, it can seem a daunting prospect.

Many successful slimmers find it less daunting if they break down their loss into "bitesize" chunks. Half a stone at a time is popular.

If you have several stones to lose, the good news is that, provided you are prepared to follow your plan, the first few stones should disappear relatively quickly.

At a heavier weight, more calories are burned doing everyday tasks. This helps to make weight loss a little speedier than average.

Normally, a 1-2lb a week loss is considered a healthy average, but at a high starting weight, provided you do not try and cut back on your Checks allowance, and provided you are choosing a wide variety of healthy foods in order to get the range of nutrients you need, don't be worried – or surprised – if your average loss is around 2-3lb a week!

When you feel down in the dumps

Instead of turning to food for comfort, why not:

- ✔ GO OUT FOR A STROLL
- ✔ STROKE YOUR PET
- ✔ LOOK OUT OF THE WINDOW AND WATCH THE WORLD GO BY
- ✔ WATCH SOMETHING FUNNY ON TELLY
- ✔ TURN ON SOME CHEERFUL MUSIC
- ✔ TALK TO SOMEBODY
- ✔ IF YOU ARE AN E-SUPPORT MEMBER, GO ONLINE
- ✔ IMMERSE YOURSELF IN A TASK
- ✔ REMEMBER THE GOOD TIMES
- ✔ TRY AND THINK OF THREE THINGS THAT COULD MAKE THE SITUATION BETTER

Over Target?

You've reached Target Weight, you're ecstatic and vow you will never again let your weight get out of hand!

One of the best ways of staying at Target is to continue to stay in touch with Scottish Slimmers, either by attending class, or with our e-support service online.

Being realistic, your Target Weight is likely to fluctuate by a couple of pounds up or down. This is normal and nothing to worry about, but if you want to stay at TW, the secret is not to allow your weight to go more than 3lb over without doing something about it.

If you find yourself 3lb or 4lb over TW, it means that you are eating a little more than you need. Check that you are not becoming too lax about portions sizes, or allowing a few too many treats to creep in. It might be that just cutting back a little will do the trick.

Or could it be that you are less active now than when you were consciously losing weight?

Of course, we allow a very generous 7lb over TW, but you should really think of this as the absolute maximum. It's not for nothing that 7lb over is known as your "danger weight"!

Alternatively, you could return to your weight loss level of Checks for a week or two until you are right back to your Target Weight, or at least within a pound or two. Having done this, you will then need to increase your Checks gradually back up to your long-term maintenance level over the next two or three weeks to give your body a chance to adjust to eating a little more.

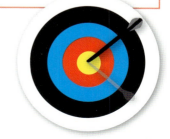

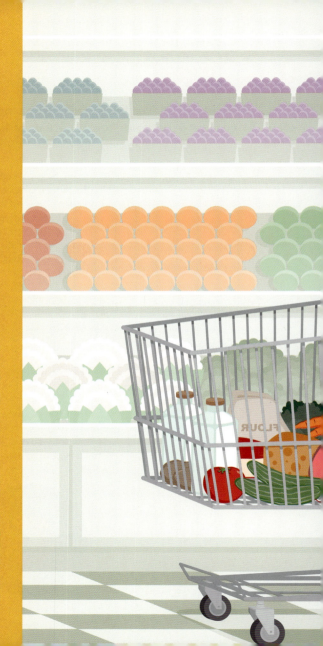

Hints on habits

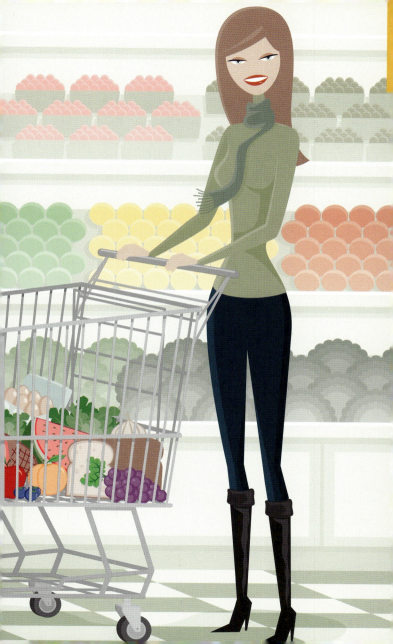

One step at a time

Most of us know that we have certain habits that are the cause of our being overweight. The secret of being slim is to recognise what these are and gradually – one step at a time – make the permanent changes necessary to eliminate old bad habits and replace them with new good habits.

In many instances we turn to food for comfort when we are emotionally upset or we eat simply because the food is there and there is no immediate reason to deny ourselves.

In the following pages we'll talk about some of the tips and tricks you can use to make small practical changes that can have a big impact, but the first step is to think about what it is that is stopping you from being slim.

Could it be any of the following?

- ✓ HAVING TOO MUCH FOOD AROUND YOU.
- ✓ EATING IN SECRET.
- ✓ HAVING TOO MANY TAKEAWAYS.
- ✓ HAVING TOO MANY HIGH-CHECK BETWEEN MEAL SNACKS.
- ✓ ABSENT-MINDEDLY PUTTING FOOD IN YOUR MOUTH.
- ✓ DRINKING TOO MUCH ALCOHOL.
- ✓ REWARDING YOURSELF (AND PROBABLY OTHERS) WITH SWEETS, CAKES, BISCUITS, ETC.
- ✓ TRYING TO DENY YOURSELF TOO STRICTLY.

In fact, it's probably more than one thing, but once you acknowledge what you do, you can start to make changes that will make a difference.

For example, if you usually have three takeaway meals a week, think of the difference it could make if you only had one a week instead.

Of course there will be many complex reasons why we have got into the habit of turning to food for comfort, but at some point we have to try and take some practical steps to break the link and set our own boundaries.

You can't change everything at once – don't even try – but do try and think about what would make a real difference and how you can, and will, make some sort of change to a behaviour that will give you a really positive outcome.

Plating up

Some slimmers say they find it helpful to serve their meals on smaller plates, so their food doesn't look lost!

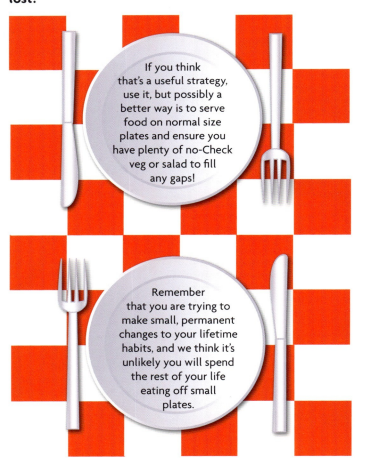

If you think that's a useful strategy, use it, but possibly a better way is to serve food on normal size plates and ensure you have plenty of no-Check veg or salad to fill any gaps!

Remember that you are trying to make small, permanent changes to your lifetime habits, and we think it's unlikely you will spend the rest of your life eating off small plates.

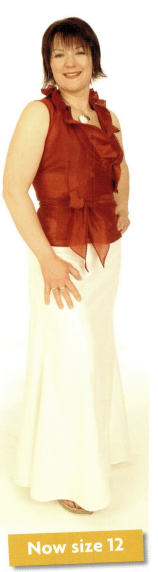

Mandy Martin

" **Variety is the spice of life – I recommend using the recipe and meal ideas in the Positive Eating Plan to avoid getting bored of the same dishes every week.** "

Weight loss:
4 stone 1 lb

Now size 12

Better in the bin

Most of us hate food waste, and it's shocking to hear of how much food we throw away as a nation — but this is essentially because we buy too much in the first place.

When it comes to leftovers, how guilty are you of eating up the odd roast potato that someone left on their plate (probably one of the kids or a skinny partner), or finishing up food that's left in pots and pans?

If there is frequently a lot of food leftover in pots and pans (and on other people's plates) you are probably cooking too much in the first place. Cook less in future, unless you are intentionally batch cooking, which is a great idea.

If you are, a good trick is to serve the amount you intend to freeze into suitable containers before serving out the meal you intend to eat immediately. It'll be job done, and nothing to pick at when it comes to washing up or stacking the dishwasher.

If you are the one that clears away a meal, get into the habit of scraping plates straight into the bin. (Some people say they squeeze a bit of washing up liquid over the leftovers before scraping into the bin — to stop them from picking and to make absolutely sure there is no going back!).

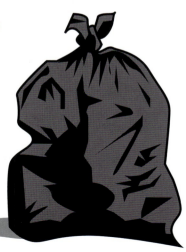

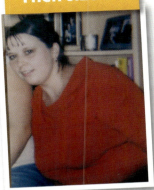

Then size 20

Vikki Armstrong

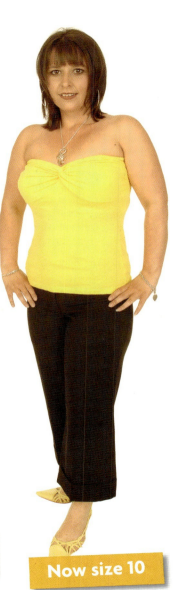

" Don't give up – every chocolate-free moment is worth it! "

Weight loss:
4 stone 6 lbs

Now size 10

Out of sight, out of mind

Seeing food is one of the main triggers for eating – especially if you are feeling a little peckish! It makes sense, therefore, to keep food stored out of sight as much as possible.

In the kitchen, keep all food in cupboards, fridge or freezer, but also give a thought to which cupboard you put things in. For example, don't store biscuits or snacks next to the tea bags or coffee jar, because you know that every time you make a cuppa you'll be tempted into an automatic snack.

If you must keep sweets in your handbag or car, it goes without saying that a few sugar-free sweets or gum are the best choices.

With the possible exception of a fruit bowl, it's best not to store food in any other room in the house.

If you are at a party, don't stand near a bowl of nuts, nor near the buffet table. You know you won't be able to resist!

And last, but not least, a reminder that it's wise to do your food shopping after you have eaten. You'll be better equipped to deal with the sight of all that food and you are much more likely to stick with your list, and less likely to devour something on the way home.

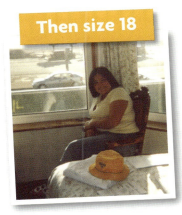

Jane McGeachy

" Write everything down you eat – it really does help you keep count of Checks. "

Weight loss:
2 stone 12 lbs

Now size 10

Slow down

Are you a fast eater? Many of us are.

Apart from the fact that it takes around 20 minutes for your stomach to send messages to your brain registering that you have eaten a meal, if you finish a meal in 10 minutes flat, psychologically you will feel short-changed.

Make every meal an occasion! Forget reading or watching television whilst eating. Try putting your knife and fork down between bites and savour each mouthful.

If you are not using a knife it could be indicative that the food you are eating is over-processed. Such foods are quick to get into your mouth and quick to swallow!

Put texture into your meals with plenty of lightly cooked veggies, or a side salad. You don't have to chew each mouthful a hundred times, but chewing thoroughly does aid digestion, especially of carbohydrate foods (which includes fruits and vegetables as well as breads, potatoes, pasta and rice). The first stage in their digestion should be the action of the enzyme amylase (in the saliva) starting the process of breaking down starches into simple sugars. But it only happens if the food is in your mouth for a few seconds and is chewed thoroughly!

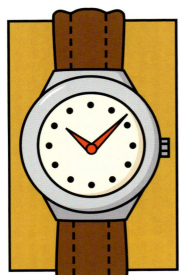

Try timing yourself to see how long it normally takes you to eat a main meal.

Trick or treat

Many slimmers will tell you that the secret of their success is their daily dose of chocolate!

Trying to permanently deny yourself your favourite foods never works (remember we are talking lifetime habits here) so it is a good idea to find an appropriate way of including them.

For some people a small daily dose is ideal. They look forward to it and are happy to stick with healthier foods the rest of the day. Choosing small packs or individually wrapped portions of your favourites can be a great help here. If this is for you, set your own personal boundary of unwrapping only one or two items a day.

But this doesn't suit everyone. If you know that once you start on something you won't be satisfied until you've had a good amount, it might be better for you to save a few Checks each day for a larger treat once or twice a week.

Even if you choose this approach it is still important to know what your boundaries are. It's probably better to buy your treat on the day you intend to eat it, and buy only in the size you have planned for if you know anything more will be difficult to resist.

Look at the label

A good way of ensuring success is to know what you are putting into your mouth!

It's so easy to make assumptions about food and often the reality doesn't match the assumption. If you are buying something new, it's best to do a little label checking.

When it comes to weight management, like it or not, the most significant factor is the energy value of a food – in other words, calories. As many products are sold in countries all around the world, the energy values are given both as k/cals, short for kilocalories, and as k/joules, short for kilojoules. In the UK we are interested in the figure for k/cals or kilocalories. (Joules are preferred in Europe, Canada and Australia.)

If a product doesn't at least have a back of pack nutrition label giving details per 100g, it's probably better to give it a miss! You could try contacting the company for the information. By law a contact name and address or telephone number or website address has to appear on the pack, but chances are that if the information isn't on the pack, the company hasn't had the food analysed (it's not a legal requirement).

Luckily most foods do now carry the information and, better still, will also give details for a stated portion of the food in addition to the values per 100g. Life gets even easier when calories per portion also appear on the front of packs. Do make sure that the portion you intend to eat matches the portion size stated, or that you double the calories if you have double the portion!

Likewise, if values are only given per 100g, you need to take into account how many grams you will be eating if it's more or less than 100g.

Equally important, take note of whether the values given are for the food as sold, or after it has been cooked according to instructions.

When you know how many calories in your portion, divide by 25 to find the number of Checks. In most instances it will make little difference if you round values to the nearest whole Check. With low value items (less than 100 calories) you may want to round to the nearest half-Check.

"Per 100g cooked" does not mean you take 100g of the product and then cook it – it is the value for 100g weight of the product after it has been cooked. With some foods this makes quite a difference!

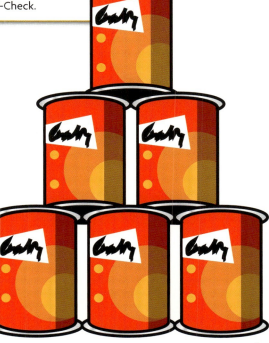

Write it down

It's not necessary to keep a note of everything you eat in order to lose weight, especially if you are selecting meals only from the PEP and perhaps adding one or two Essential Extras, but writing down everything you eat has more benefits than simply keeping a tally on the number of Checks you have spent.

FIRSTLY, IT TENDS TO KEEP YOUR MIND FOCUSED ON THE JOB IN HAND.

If you are making up your own recipes and menus and adding essential extras, it will keep you within your checks allowance, but always try and write things down as you eat them – if you leave it to the end of the day and try and remember what you've had, you're sure to forget something!

YOU CAN KEEP A NOTE OF YOUR FAT GRAM INTAKE ALSO.

YOU CAN KEEP TRACK OF YOUR EVERY DAY BONUS FOODS – DO YOU REALLY HAVE 6-8 GLASSES OF FLUIDS EVERY DAY?

IT CAN HELP YOU SPOT IF YOU ARE SPENDING TOO MANY CHECKS ON TREAT FOODS AND NOT ENOUGH ON NUTRITIOUS FOODS.

YOU CAN ALSO ADD COMMENTS ABOUT HOW YOU FEEL ON ANY GIVEN DAY, OR WHETHER OR NOT YOU PARTICULARLY ENJOYED A MEAL.

YOU CAN KEEP A NOTE OF HOW MUCH EXERCISE YOU DO EACH DAY (OR NOT!).

IF YOU KEEP ALL THAT YOU'VE WRITTEN, YOU CAN USE PAST SHEETS TO HELP YOU PLAN ANOTHER WEEK'S MENUS.

YOU MIGHT BE ABLE TO SPOT PATTERNS IN YOUR EATING BEHAVIOUR.

YOU CAN REPEAT A WEEK WHEN YOU HAD A GOOD WEIGHT LOSS.

By writing everything down you can gain a lot of valuable information about yourself and your eating behaviours, but it is only worth the paper it's written on if it's the truth, the whole truth and nothing but the truth!

Stay out of the danger zones

The kitchen

Of course you can't avoid going into the kitchen completely, but you know that's where most of your food is stored (hopefully, out of sight in cupboards, fridge or freezer) and, especially if you are at home all day — and many of us are at weekends if not during the week — it's all too easy to help ourselves to something we really don't need.

Being in the kitchen for food preparation, cooking and washing up is fine — but if you happen to feel a little bit bored and a little bit hungry, what is likely to happen if you wander into the kitchen?

Food shops

We all have to go into them but many of us find it very difficult to come out with only the one thing we went in to buy!

Try and keep food shopping trips to the minimum, which is best done by planning your weekly menu ahead of time.

Plan to have fresh and chilled foods at the start of your shopping week (things that are likely to have a "use before" date), and use frozen and storecupboard goods towards the end.

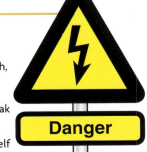

Cafés and Coffee Shops

If you are happy to have just a skinny latte, go ahead. For most of us, though, the sight of those over-sized muffins, filled baguettes, panninis and other goodies can turn a relaxing coffee break into a shall I? shan't I? nightmare.

The moral is simply — don't put yourself under needless pressure.

Delay tactics

It could be that it's getting near to a meal time and you are starting to feel hungry, or perhaps you just fancy eating something for no particular reason.

Here are three tips that many successful slimmers use to get them through such a moment.

1 Sip a glass of water

It's surprising how a glass of water can tie you over for a little while. In cold weather, a cup of hot water does the trick for some people.   It is also true that we frequently mistake thirst for hunger in which case the water satisfies the need.

2 Wait 10 minutes

Make yourself wait 10 minutes before you eat anything. Try and do something constructive in those 10 minutes such as making a phone call, write out a 'to do' list, empty the dishwasher. More often than not, you get engrossed in what you are doing and the urge passes.

3 Go clean your teeth

Eating just doesn't seem right with that fresh minty taste in your mouth! Incidentally, it's also worth remembering that your teeth come under attack from acid for about 20 minutes after every time you eat. If you keep popping things in your mouth continually throughout the day, you could be damaging your teeth as well as your waistline.

Vary your diet

There are two great reasons for varying your diet.

Firstly, variety prevents boredom. If you intend sticking with an eating plan for any length of time, you certainly don't want to get bored with it.

How many different meals have you tried from the PEP? Why not aim to try out something new at least once a week?

You can get even more ideas from our cook books (available in class or on line). All recipes are Check and fat gram counted to make them easy to fit into your plan and they cover a wide range of themes from very simple to prepare to something more special. And you don't need to be an expert cook to get great results!

The other important reason for including a good variety of foods is to ensure you get the full range of nutrients you need for good health.

EACH DAY YOU NEED FOODS FROM EACH OF THE FOUR MAIN FOOD GROUPS:

FRUIT AND VEGETABLES

BREADS, CEREALS, POTATOES, PASTA, RICE AND OTHER STARCHY GRAINS AND VEGETABLES

MEAT, FISH, EGGS, PULSES OR VEGETARIAN ALTERNATIVES

MILK, LOW-FAT DAIRY FOODS OR OTHER HIGH-CALCIUM ALTERNATIVES

Foods containing a lot of fat or sugar or alcohol are enjoyable and something to look forward to but are best kept as "treats" as they frequently have a high Check value and if they take up too large a proportion of your Check allowance, it will mean that you are not eating enough of the healthier, nutrient-dense foods.

The different colours of fruits and veg indicate the presence of different nutrients many of which have a protective antioxidant effect.

As well as providing energy, breads and cereals made from different grains such as wheat, oats, rye and rice provide different types of fibre, some which help lower cholesterol levels, others keep the digestive tract working efficiently.

Meat, fish and alternatives provide the protein necessary for repair of every cell in the body and is required for growth in children and pregnant women. Vegetarians in particular should use a variety of vegetarian protein foods in order to get the range of amino acids required to make the type of complete proteins required by the body.

Although all dairy foods supply good amounts of calcium some, such as cheese, are high in salt, so it would be unwise to rely solely on cheese as a source of calcium.

Be prepared!

Like it or not, hunger will strike – and if you're not prepared for it, you'll likely devour the first thing you see!

Have you ever found yourself in that situation where you come home tired and hungry and realise you've planned to have a casserole for dinner that's going to take two hours to cook.

No chance. You have to be realistic if you want to be successful.

When you are planning your meals and snacks for the week, think about when you are going to eat them as well as what you are going to eat.

Write out a schedule of when are the best times for you to eat. Weekends might be different from workdays.

Do all you can to have food ready to eat at those times.

- Are there things you could prepare in advance in order to reduce the time it takes to get a meal on the table?
- **Each morning try and remember if you need to take anything out of the freezer to defrost.**
- Batch cook whenever you can and freeze in portions for another day.
- **A portion of frozen rice can be microwaved in a couple of minutes.**
- Have one or two ready meals in the freezer for very busy days.
- **Prepare packed lunches the night before.**
- Keep a carton of longlife skimmed milk in the cupboard in case you run out of fresh.
- **Keep an apple nearby – it's very portable and can count as one of your Every Day Bonus fruits (or if you have already had your two average servings of fruit, it will only cost you 2 Checks).**
- Ready-prepared packs of stir-fry veg and salad leaves save peeling, chopping and washing time.
- **Make the most of your microwave. Microwave cooking is very healthy as the shorter cooking time preserves vitamins.**

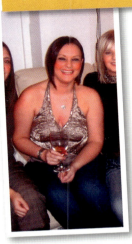

Laura Gallagher

" Don't skip breakfast – make sure it's one of your three meals a day. "

Weight loss:
2 stone 4 lbs

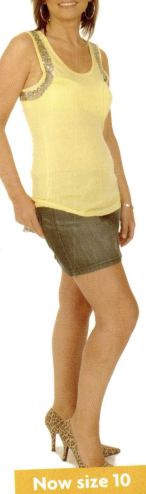

Now size 10

Sleep and slim!

Getting sufficient sleep is a great aid to weight loss!

We don't mean that fat will magically disappear when asleep (although we do burn around 50-60 calories an hour), but getting sufficient sleep means we can get through the day with more vim and vigour.

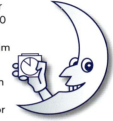

The amount of sleep needed varies from person to person. A very few people function well on just four hours sleep a night, some need eight or nine hours, but the majority of us need around seven hours.

If we've had enough sleep, we can do everything at a reasonable pace, and can get through more tasks in a day than if we feel tired and lethargic. Doing more means burning more calories.

If we burn just an extra 10 calories per hour for around 13-14 of our waking hours each day we could burn off around an extra 49,000 calories a year. At roughly 3,500 calories per pound of fat, those 49,000 calories equate to 1 stone!

In order to burn more calories per hour, try:

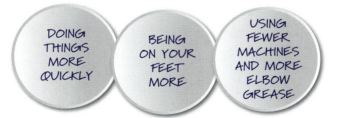

DOING THINGS MORE QUICKLY

BEING ON YOUR FEET MORE

USING FEWER MACHINES AND MORE ELBOW GREASE

Of course, the other advantage of getting more sleep is that whilst you are asleep, you can't eat!

Get a life!

Many people make the mistake of putting their life on hold until they reach Target Weight assuming that once they are slim, everything else in their life will be wonderful.

There's no doubt that being slim makes you feel physically so much better and, more often than not, psychologically gives you the confidence to dare to do things you never would before.

But there's no need to wait until you are slim to start enjoying life.

Think about acquiring a new skill or qualification that could perhaps put you in line for promotion at work.

Take up a new hobby or interest, so you have something other than food to talk about.

Take an interest in other people and go out with them every so often. Visit a cinema, theatre, concert, museum, have a leisurely walk in the country or by the sea, enjoy a social gathering. If food is involved, it's a chance to practice what you have learned about eating moderate portions and choosing healthier foods whenever you can. You'll need these skills when you are slim — if you wish to stay slim!

Occupational therapy

Many of us spend too much time watching television and, more often than not, that involves snacking.

Why not turn off the box and get involved in something else. Here are a dozen suggestions:

RESEARCH YOUR FAMILY TREE.

TRY BRAIN TRAINING — YOU DON'T HAVE TO HAVE THAT FAMOUS HANDHELD MACHINE, AS MAGAZINES ARE AVAILABLE.

GIVE YOURSELF A MANICURE OR PEDICURE.

READ A GOOD BOOK.

BROWSE THROUGH CATALOGUES.

MAKE GREETINGS CARDS - HANDMADE CARDS ARE SO IN!

RESTORE A PIECE OF FURNITURE.

KNIT A SWEATER.

EMBROIDER AN HEIRLOOM.

SORT OUT A DRAWER — IT'S AMAZING WHAT YOU FIND AND HOW GOOD YOU FEEL WHEN IT'S DONE!

DO A CROSSWORD OR SUDOKU OR WORDSEARCH.

WRITE A POEM.

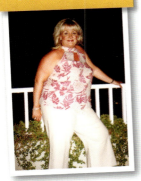

Hazel Johnston Cranna

" **My Check book is my bible – I take it everywhere I go.** "

Weight loss:
5 stone 3 lbs

Now size 12

Perfect week

Have you ever had a perfect week when you haven't cheated once on your eating plan? Quite an achievement if you have!

How about going for it this week?

Get yourself a length of string.

At the end of each day, if you feel you have followed your plan perfectly, tie a knot in the string.

The aim is to have seven knots in your string by the end of the week.

Tough? Yes, but we reckon that many people can easily manage five or six knots, and if you do achieve seven, we bet you'll end the week with a fantastic weight loss!

Don't give up too easily

Many of us have lost several stones in our lifetime – the trouble is we frequently lose – and then regain – the same couple of stones over and over again!

Most people give up because they are not happy with their progress, but they forget that making progress requires making permanent changes.

✔ It means that you really are trying to eat more healthily most of the time, not just when you are trying to lose weight.

✔ It means learning to draw a line under the occasional bad day or three, and getting straight back to your plan.

✔ It means that it is still worth sticking to your plan for the next few days even though you know you will be having a celebration meal at the weekend.

✔ It means that should you have a disappointment at the scales, you don't blame the scales, but instead think about how you could improve the situation.

Weight loss rarely goes as smoothly as clockwork, but if we give up every time we have a little set back, we will never reach our destination.

Just say no!

Like it or not, sometimes the answer is simply to show a bit of restraint – and just say:

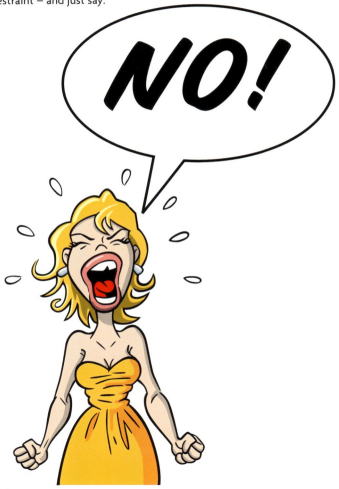

Include some easy-to-eat fruits such as apples or pears which won't make a big dent in your Check allowance should you want to nibble on something to while away the time (especially if they come out of your Every Day Bonus allowance). Some sugar-free sweets might also be useful, but remember that eating an excessive amount of these can have a laxative effect!

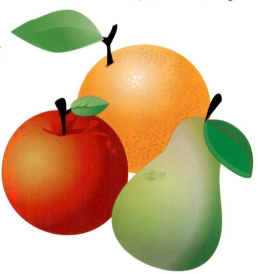

Holidays abroad

Holiday weight gain is not inevitable!

Here are some of the best tips for ensuring you don't come back with excess baggage!

From the outset decide that, even if you allow yourself a few extra treats, you will generally keep things under control.

Have one special meal a day when you choose whatever you fancy – but in moderate portions.

Choose wisely from buffets – and only fill your plate once.

Keep other meals or snacks relatively small and/or low-Check. Make the most of local fresh fruit.

Fish and poultry dishes are likely to be better choices than meat dishes.

If possible, avoid sauces made from butter, cheese or cream. If salads are already dressed with oil, leave as much oil as possible on the plate!

Enjoy a few extra treats – try a local speciality, or an ice cream, or a tempting pastry or dessert. But it doesn't have to be every day!

If sugar-free drinks are not easily available, go for bottled water.

Plan to be more active than usual – you'll have more time to walk, more time to swim, more time to play with the kids, more time to dance the night away.

Limit yourself to no more than 2 alcoholic drinks a day – well, you did want to come back without a weight gain, didn't you!

School holidays

Why is it that weight loss seems more difficult when the children are off school?

Firstly, our usual routine becomes disrupted.

You know it's going to happen, so you need to prepare for a different routine. It's not a bad idea to try to do some batch cooking and freezing in advance, to save time and effort when you need to. Also, decide in advance whether you will have your main meal with the children. If not, it's a good idea to plan to have a snack with them when they have theirs, rather than sit down with them and pinch the chips off their plate or eat up all their leftovers!

If you take the kids out, you might frequently find yourself in fast-food restaurants.

Many now offer healthier alternatives (for you and the children!). Alternatively, pack-up your own food to take and try to get the children to help in the preparation. Think rolls, wraps, low-fat crisps, no-added sugar drinks, low-fat cake slices and plenty of fruit.

If the kids play up, we become more stressed out.

Again, it's probably worth the effort of a bit of advance planning to arrange some activities for the kids to take part in. You could have a "good behaviour chart" awarding points or stars with appropriate prizes for the number of points or stars gained each week. And if you know other mums with children, try sharing the kids around so that you can all have a bit of a break in turns!

Invitation to dinner

Your friend, who is a fantastic cook, has asked you over for dinner – and you know she is going to spend hours cooking for you and it will be so delicious that it's going to be hard to resist!

At the time of the invitation, why not just mention to her that you'd love to come but (as she may well know) you've been losing weight and eating much more healthily of late, so there's no need to go to a lot of trouble – something light and simple would be fantastic.

Demonstrate your commitment to a healthier lifestyle by giving your hostess flowers rather than a box of chocolates!

If, however, her idea of something light is not your idea of something light, then try and make the best of the situation.

DON'T start on nuts or crisps with pre-dinner drinks.

PASS on bread rolls, or bread and dipping oil.

TRY to have modest portions or just a taster of everything.

IF it's all served on the plate in the modern style, don't be afraid to leave a little on the plate.

IF you've had a dessert, avoid cheese and biscuits if they are also on offer – she didn't spend hours cooking those!

IF you compliment her on how delicious the food is, she probably won't even notice how much or how little you have eaten.

What's your weight in kilos?

Most of us think of our weight only in stones and pounds, but it's a good idea to get to know what your Target Weight is, or will be, in kilograms. Knowing this is one of the secrets of staying slim.

Find your Target Weight (or the nearest to it) on the chart below and note what it is in kilograms.

st lb	kgs	st lb	kgs
7 12	50	12 02	77
8 03	52	12 08	80
8 09	55	12 13	82
9 00	57	13 05	85
9 06	60	13 10	87
9 11	62	14 02	90
10 03	65	14 07	92
10 08	67	14 13	95
11 00	70	15 04	97
11 05	72	15 10	100
11 11	75		

Your Target Weight in kilograms will be the approximate number of Checks you can have on average each day in order to maintain your Target Weight in the long term. Men should be able to add up to a further 10 Checks a day.

Your lifestyle, age and usual level of activity affect your energy needs, so it may be necessary to do a bit of fine-tuning to find exactly the right amount for you.

When you have reached TW, you won't be able to go onto this maintenance level of Checks immediately. It will take a few weeks to gradually work up from your weight loss level of Checks to this maintenance level.

However, it's always a good thing to keep in mind that if you want to keep your weight at, say, 70 kilos, then 70 Checks a day is about the average you need to stick with – but you can still have your Every Day Bonus foods on top!

You are what you eat a lot of!

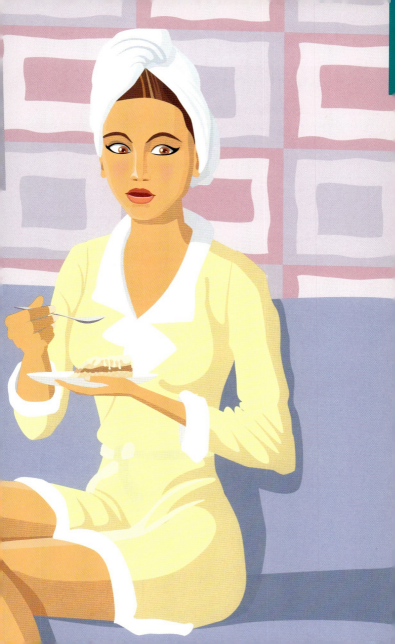

Water, water everywhere

Many successful slimmers tell us that they feel good and find it much easier to stick to their plan when they ensure they have their 6-8 glasses of water or fluids every day.

Although tea and coffee do have some diuretic effect, they do still count, as you do not lose all that you have drunk.

It is really important to ensure you drink sufficient fluids each day. Around 60% of our total body weight is water and is used in many vital systems such as transporting nutrients around the body, as a lubricant and in the regulation of body temperature.

Symptoms of dehydration such as headaches, muscle cramps, dizziness, faintness, start to occur when we lose just 2% of our water.

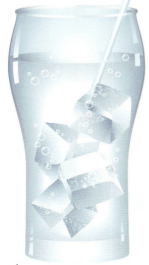

It is very important for athletes, or anyone working out in a gym or training or taking part in an event to keep well hydrated and to remember that they will need more than 8 glasses a day.

Dark gold urine is a sign of dehydration. It should be a pale straw colour if you are well hydrated.

Switch 'n' save

Switching to lower-fat, lower-Check foods doesn't always make a huge difference on one single item, but over a day it can make a big difference.

The table below shows items that could easily be eaten on a typical day and compares them with better choice items.

Saving a few Checks here and there really can make a difference!

Typical Food	Checks	Better Food	Checks	Checks Saved
2 thick slices bread	8	2 medium slices bread	6	**2**
10g butter	3	10g low-fat spread	1.5	**1.5**
2 tsp marmalade	2	2 tsp reduced-sugar marmalade	1	**1**
300ml semi-skimmed milk	5	300ml skimmed milk	4	**1**
30g cheddar	5	30g half-fat cheddar	3	**2**
Individual chicken pie	18	Oven-baked breaded chicken breast	11	**7**
150g home-made chips	12	150g low-fat oven chips	9	**3**
150g Muller Amoré Yoghurt	9	200g Mullerlight Yoghurt	4	**5**
2 x 60ml scoops luxury ice cream	12	2 x 60ml regular plain ice cream	4	**8**
Alpen cereal bar	5	Alpen Light cereal bar	2.5	**2.5**
330ml can of fizzy drink	6	330ml can diet fizzy drink	0	**6**
Total Checks	85	Total Checks	46	**39**

Where's the fat?

If you wish to keep down your total intake of fat, these are the foods you need to be very careful about, especially if eaten in large quantities:

Food	Approx. grams of fat in 100g
Oil, all types	100
Lard, white fats and ghee	100
Suet (beef or vegetable)	87
Butter	80
Macadamia nuts	78
Brazil nuts, pecans, pine nuts, walnuts	70
Creamed coconut	70
Hazelnuts	65
Desiccated coconut	60
Reduced fat spreads	60
Almonds, cashew nuts, peanuts, pistachios	50-55
Peanut butter	50
Pumpkin seeds, sunflower seeds	45-50
Double cream	45
Cream cheese, full fat	45
Pork scratchings or crackling	45
Chicken skin, roasted	45
Whipping cream	40
Crème fraîche, full fat	40
Roast duck with fat and skin	40
Crisps	35
Chocolate	35
Chocolate spread	35
Hard cheeses and Stilton, full fat	35

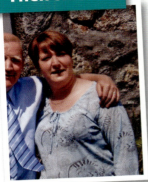

Jill Philip

❝ I set myself small targets – and only talked about target when I had lost the first five stone! ❞

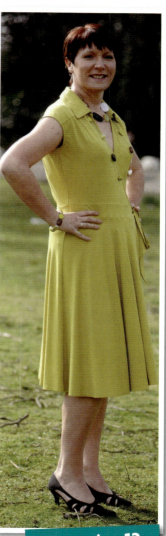

Weight loss:
6 stone

Now size 12

Where's the sugar?

For good health – and for the protection of our teeth – we are advised not to eat too much sugar. There are many different types of sugars and we do not need to be concerned about the amounts found naturally in fruits and vegetables (mostly fructose), nor that found naturally in milk and dairy products (lactose).

We should aim to have no more than 90g a day of sugars in total, but the ones we should be most careful about are those which have been added to food products. Looking at the ingredients list on a label will tell you if sugar has been added. As ingredients are listed with most first, be wary if sugar is listed in the first two or three ingredients.

As well as looking for words such as sugar, honey and syrup, also look out for other types of sugar that frequently end in "ose" such as sucrose, glucose, dextrose, maltose.

Food	Approx. grams of sugar in 100g
Sugar	100
Peppermints	100
Boiled sweets	85
Golden syrup	80
Fudge	80
Honey	75
Jam and marmalade	70
Turkish delight	70
Marshmallows	65
Treacle	65
Marzipan	65
Chocolate	60
Chocolate spread or chocolate & nut spread	60
Mincemeat (sweet)	60
Gums and jelly sweets	60
Jaffa cakes	55
Chocolate cakes, iced cakes and fruit cakes	45-55
Sugar or honey coated breakfast cereals	40-50
Toffees	45
Wafer biscuits	45
Cream-filled biscuits	35-40
Sweet biscuits including chocolate coated	30-35
Plain cakes and teabreads	30-35
Cereal bars	30
Sweet & sour sauce	30
Semi-sweet biscuits	25

Where's the salt?

Too much salt is bad for your blood pressure and will also make you retain fluid that can show up as a gain on the scales.

We should be aiming to have no more than 6g of salt a day, which is just a bit more than 1 teaspoon. Most of the salt we eat comes from pre-packed processed foods and ready meals, especially those that are not part of a "healthy" range, but many manufacturers have already made some reductions and are looking to make more. You need to check the label as brands vary considerably.

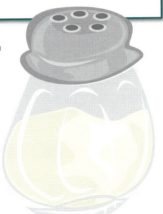

Ideally, we should prepare as much of our own food as possible using fresh ingredients so that we can control the amount of salt that is added, but even here we need to take care.

Food	Approx. grams of salt in portion
1 tsp salt	5
150g raw weight gammon rasher	5
10g stock cube (e.g. Knorr)	4
6g stock cube (e.g. Oxo)	2.25
1 tsp bouillon powder (e.g. Marigold)	2.25
50g smoked salmon	2.25
300g can of soup	2
200g can steak in gravy	2
1 tsp Lo-Salt	1.75
1 dspn soy sauce	1.75
125g pasta sauce	0.5-1.25
2 slices Parma ham	1.25
30g smoked bacon	1.25
30g unsmoked bacon	1
30g ham	1
1 rounded tsp yeast extract (e.g. Marmite)	1
1 tsp baking powder	1
1 large pork sausage	1
30g corned beef	0.75
30g cornflakes	0.75
1 dspn instant gravy granules	0.75
30g vacuum-pack chicken breast	0.5
1 medium slice bread	0.5
1 tbsp tomato ketchup or brown sauce	0.5
25g pack of crisps	0.5
30g hard cheese	0.5
1 tbsp low-calorie mayonnaise	0.3-0.5

Make it easy on yourself

We're all busy these days so it's no wonder many of us want to cook express meals like Nigella or cheat like Delia. Well, we're all for the easy life, but you need to be a little careful about products you choose.

Some really useful products are:

Frozen vegetables

These are equally as high in vitamins and minerals as fresh. Our online members seem to agree that some of the most useful are sliced or chopped onions, sliced or chopped peppers, sliced mushrooms. Carrots and swede are useful for casseroles, stews and soups. Even top celebrity chefs agree that frozen peas are really hard to beat. Individual packs of micro-steam veg are very useful if you are cooking for one.

Stir-fry vegetables

Pre-prepared packs of fresh chopped stir-fry vegetables save time and often save money and waste over buying individual items. You can usually find packs that comprise only no-Check veg such as beansprouts, greens, onions, peppers, carrot, mushrooms. Don't be too concerned if they contain a little sweetcorn. The amount in one serving is unlikely to exceed a tablespoon, so you only need to count 1 Check.

Prepared salad leaves
Enough said!

Chillies, garlic and ginger

EPC Very Lazy Chillies, Garlic or Ginger may be used freely. Dried chilli flakes also pack a punch and save chopping chillies. Garlic or ginger in sunflower oil, such as Bart Spices, work out at about 1 Check for a heaped teaspoon, which is probably enough for 2-4 servings, so is well worth the time you save in peeling, crushing or grating.

Potatoes

If you hate peeling then jacket potatoes or new potatoes are the answer. Don't forget you can microwave jacket potatoes and then, if you have time, you can crisp up the skin in a hot oven for 10 minutes. You can also microwave them, cut into wedges, spritz with a few sprays of oil and bake in a hot oven for yummy wedges. Low-fat oven chips are easier and lower-Check than homemade, but can take quite a while to crisp up if you are cooking for more than one person.

Pulses and lentils

Canned pulses and lentils such as chickpeas and kidney beans save hours of soaking and boiling time over dried, but you should look out for those that have no salt added. Most major supermarkets are now gradually switching over to no-added-salt varieties if they have not already done so.

Lean meat

Buying "healthy" range fresh meats saves trimming but usually comes at a premium price. However, as there is virtually no waste, it may not be as expensive as you first think.

Skinless & boneless canned fish

If you don't like skin and bones, these save lots of fiddling around time. We particularly like Glenryk's Skinless & Boneless Medium Red Salmon and Tesco's Skinless & Boneless Wild Pacific Pink Salmon.

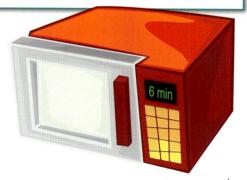

The eye of the beholder

A good idea that helps many a slimmer is to make food look really satisfying. There are several little tricks you can use.

GRATE CHEESE FINELY FOR SALADS, SANDWICHES OR PIZZA TOPPINGS. IT MAKES A LITTLE GO A LOT FURTHER.

CUT NEW POTATOES IN HALF – YOU'LL FEEL AS THOUGH YOU HAVE TWICE AS MANY!!

CHOOSE THINNER STEAKS AND CHOPS – THEY'LL TAKE UP MORE ROOM ON THE PLATE.

✔ CUT AN APPLE INTO WEDGES AND ARRANGE ON A PLATE. IN COLD WEATHER YOU CAN SPRINKLE THE WEDGES WITH A LITTLE BIT OF SPICE AND POP IN THE MICROWAVE FOR A MINUTE OR TWO TO TURN YOUR APPLE INTO A DESSERT. ALSO WORKS WELL WITH PEARS.

✔ SOME PEOPLE LIKE TO ALLOCATE A SPECIFIC NUMBER OF CHECKS EACH WEEK FOR SNACKS AND TREATS SUCH AS CRISPS, CEREAL BARS, BISCUITS OR SWEETS. THEY THEN PUT A SELECTION OF ITEMS UP TO THAT CHECK VALUE INTO A SUITABLE CONTAINER. THEY CAN THEN PICK AND CHOOSE ITEMS THROUGHOUT THE WEEK BUT KNOW THAT WHEN THEY'RE GONE, THEY'RE GONE!

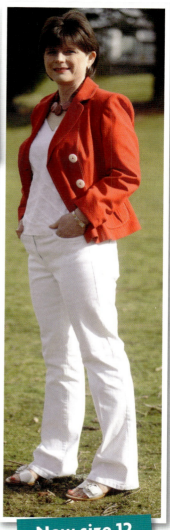

Then size 16

Arlene Deans

" I rediscovered a joy of cooking which I had lost, and my children are delighted they are getting delicious meals again. "

Weight loss: 4 stone 12 lbs

Now size 12

Soup it up

Scottish slimmers love soup – especially No-Check varieties!

Being able to have something warming, delicious and filling that you don't have to count from your Checks allowance is what has kept many on the straight and narrow.

One word of caution is to add as little as possible in the way of salt or stock or you could be having too much salt. Gradually reduce the amount you use and increase the amount of herbs and spices for extra flavour. Fortunately, the amount of veggies used in many No-Check soups contain quite a lot of potassium which helps to balance out the sodium in salt.

Our famous Technicolour Soup contains a good variety of different coloured vegetables and has no added salt.

Technicolour Soup

2 onions, peeled and chopped

2 cloves garlic, peeled and chopped

2 large carrots, peeled and sliced

2 large sticks celery, sliced

3-4 "chunks" frozen spinach or about 8 small florets fresh or frozen broccoli

2 x 400g cans tomatoes

2 tbsp tomato purée

Put all ingredients in a large saucepan, breaking up the tomatoes. Add as much or as little water as you like.

Bring to the boil, cover, reduce heat and simmer until vegetables are tender.

Start with a salad

A good way to make a meal even more filling is to have a no-Check salad as a starter.

Having raw veg often means precious vitamins are not lost in cooking – although some nutrients become more available to the body when they have been cooked, so enjoy both raw and cooked veg!

How about trying one of these for a change – they are made entirely from no-Check foods:

Carrot, beetroot & cucumber salad

Arrange a few torn romaine or little gem lettuce leaves on a plate. Coarsely grate 1 carrot and scatter over the leaves. Chop 1 cooked beetroot (not in vinegar) and a chunk of cucumber and put on top of the carrot. Squeeze over some lemon or lime juice and black pepper.

Courgette & cherry tomato salad

Thinly slice some courgette, 1 small spring onion and halve 3-4 cherry tomatoes. Toss in a little balsamic vinegar. Arrange some rocket or other salad leaves on a plate. Scatter with the courgette, onion and tomatoes. If you can, make this in advance and leave the veg to marinate in the balsamic vinegar a few hours or overnight before arranging on the salad leaves.

Stirring stuff

The beauty of stir-fries is that you can have a variety of veg with only one pan to wash up!

Stir-fries don't always have to be a complete meal — you can make interesting vegetable mixes to add to a meal, and they are absolutely ideal for using up odd bits of veg.

Red onion, tomato & kale stir-fry

Serves 2-3

Per serving: No-Check Food

Spray a pan or wok with oil and heat. Cook 1 thinly sliced red onion gently for a few minutes until starting to soften. Add 2 roughly chopped tomatoes and cook 1 minute. Add about 100g chopped kale leaves with 3-4 tbsp water. Stir-fry about 4 minutes until the water has evaporated and the leaves have wilted. (Look out for bags of ready-washed and chopped kale.)

Green bean, pepper and spring onion stir-fry

Serves 2

Per serving: No-Check Food

Spray a pan or wok with oil and heat. Add 115-150g of frozen very fine whole green beans, 4 sliced spring onions and half a large yellow or orange pepper cut into fine strips. Stir-fry about 3 minutes until crisp tender.

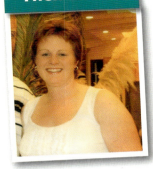

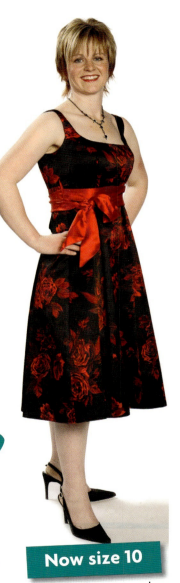

Nikki Morgan

" Encourage someone you love to give you an incentive! My partner promised me £200 to spend on clothes – and when I hit target he was happy to pay up! "

Weight loss:
3 stone 6 lbs

Now size 10

Freeze!

Snacks take longer to eat when they are frozen.

Freeze grapes in 85g/3oz portions. 1 portion can either be one of your Every Day Bonus servings of fruit, or if you have already eaten your two Every Day Bonus servings of fruit, a portion will cost you just 2 Checks.

Peel a medium banana, cut into chunks and freeze. A medium banana counts as two Every Day Bonus servings of fruit, but if taken out one chunk at a time, takes quite a while to get through.

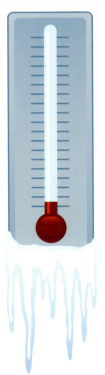

If you've got some lolly moulds, you can make no-Check lollies using diet squashes.

Slicing up a Mars or Milky Way bar seems to make it go further, but each piece will take even longer to chew if it's frozen.

Or you can make up a sachet of low-calorie chocolate drink. Let it cool and pour into lolly moulds. Many which have around 39-40 calories per sachet count as only 1½ Checks from which you can make 4-6 lollies.

It's not particularly recommended that you freeze virtually-fat-free yoghurts if you then want to eat them after defrosting, as the texture is not as good. But, if you freeze them and eat them frozen, they make a delicious, long lasting dessert. You will, however, need to take them out about 10 minutes or so before eating, because they do go rock solid!

Safe servings

We've already mentioned that individually wrapped portions of treat foods are helpful – for example, it's easier to stop at one or two individually wrapped small packets of crisps than it is to stop dipping into a 150g large bag.

But it's not only treat foods that are sold in units. Other pre-portioned foods that come in standard weights or portion sizes can help us ensure we are not having more than we should. And with some foods, it's a good idea to portion them out before starting on a new pack.

Sliced bread is not as tempting as fresh crusty bread but a slice is a slice and is likely to weigh a lot less than our attempts at cutting a medium slice from a fresh new loaf.

If ever you bake a large cake or tea loaf, cut into slices and individually wrap and freeze any that are not required immediately.

If you like cheese spread, low-fat triangles will help you stay in control more easily than dipping your knife into a tub. With low-fat or extra-light soft cheese, this frequently comes in 200g or 300g rectangular tubs. When you open a tub, it's a good idea to score the surface into 25g portions with a knife (8 portions in a 200g tub, 12 in a 300g tub).

You can do a similar scoring job with ice cream. 125ml is the equivalent of about 2 level scoops, so a 500ml tub should give you 4 x 125ml portions, 750ml tub is 6 portions, 1000ml or 1 litre tub is 8 portions and a 2 litre tub can be marked out into 16 x 2 level scoop portions.

More bang for your bucks

Research seems to indicate that we tend to eat the same volume of food each day irrespective of whether the food is high or low in calories.

Foods with a high water content, such as vegetables, are very low in calories because the water content doesn't contain any calories! This makes them a good choice when it comes to eating large amounts.

Dry foods such as biscuits, sugar, cereals and uncooked pasta and rice have a relatively higher calorie count because most of their weight is from calorie-providing nutrients such as protein and carbohydrate, which contain 4 calories per gram. Fat has a high calorie count at 9 calories per gram and does not mix well with water, so foods with a high fat content can have a very high calorie count indeed.

The table opposite gives the approximate weight that you could have for 4 Checks (100 calories) of various types of food. You'll see that for some types of food (especially fatty and dry foods) you get a very small amount whereas for others (with a high water content) you get a nice, filling amount.

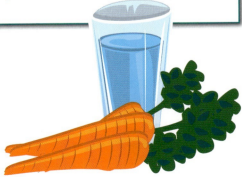

Food	What you get for 4 Checks (100 calories)
Oils	11g
Butter	13g
Nuts and seeds	15g
Chocolate	19g
Crisps	19g
Pastry, cooked	19g
Double cream	20g
Sweet biscuits	22g
Hard cheese	23g
Sugar	25g
Cakes	25g
Half-fat spread	27g
Pasta and rice (dry weight)	29g (dry weight)
Breakfast cereals	29g
Fatty meat, cooked	33g
Half-fat cheese	36g
Breads	40g
Oily fish, cooked	50g
Well-trimmed meat, cooked	57g
Skinless poultry, cooked	66g
Pasta and rice (boiled weight)	70g (boiled weight)
White fish	100g
Pulses and lentils, cooked	100g
Potatoes	143g
Fruits (average for different types)	250g
Vegetables (average for different types – but you don't need to count the Checks if they are on the no-Check list).	400g

Know what's low

It's a good idea to become familiar with foods that are the lowest Check within each type. It makes it easier to put together your own recipes and meal ideas, and you'll know what to look out for on a restaurant menu.

Fish & seafood	Checks	Fat g
Cod Fillet, raw, 100g	3	1
Coley Fillet, raw, 100g	3	1
Crab, 1 small whole, 150g in shell	3	3
Crab White Meat, 100g can, drained	2	0.5
Haddock Fillet, raw, 100g	3	1
Mixed Seafood, raw, 100g	3	0.5
Monkfish, raw, 100g	2.5	0.5
Mussels, raw in shell, 100g	1	0
Plaice Fillet, raw, 100g	3	1.5
Pollack Fillet, raw, 100g	3	0.5
Prawns, peeled, cooked, 100g	4	1
Prawns, unpeeled, cooked, 100g	2	0.5
Seafood Sticks, 2	1	0
Tuna in Brine or Water, 100g can, drained	3	1
Whiting Fillet, raw, 100g	3	1

Meat & poultry	Checks	Fat g
Bacon Medallion, grilled, 1 average	1	1
Beef Cubes, extra lean, raw, 100g	5	4
Beef Mince, less than 5% fat, raw, 100g	5	5
Beef Rump Steak, well trimmed, raw 100g	5	4
Chicken Breast, skinless, raw, 100g	4	1.5
Chicken Livers, raw, 100g	4	2.5
Ham, 15% added water, 100g	4	4
Kidney, average of all types, raw 100g	4	2.5
Lamb Leg Steaks, extra lean, raw, 100g	5	5
Pork Escalopes, raw, 100g	4	2
Pork Leg, raw, 100g	4	2
Pork Mince, less than 5% fat, raw, 100g	4	3
Proscuitto, average 12-15g slice, e.g. Parma ham	1.5	1.5
Sausage, very low fat up to 70 calories, e.g. Wall's Lean Recipe	3	2.5
Turkey Breast, skinless, raw, 100g	4	1
Turkey Dark Meat, skinless, raw, 100g	4	2.5
Turkey Rasher, grilled, 1 average	1	0.5
Veal Escalopes, raw, 100g	4	2
Venison Steak, raw, 100g	4	1.5
Wafer-thin cooked meats, e.g. chicken, ham, turkey, 2 slices	1	1

Know what's low (cont'd)

Values for branded products may change from time to time due to recipe changes, but the following are typical.

Vegetarian	Checks	Fat g
Asda Meatfree Mince, frozen, 100g	4	3
Birds Eye Soya Beans, frozen, 100g	6	6
Cauldren Foods Falafel, each	2	2.5
Cauldren Foods Lincolnshire Veggie Sausage, each	3	5
Cauldren Foods Mushroom Burger	5	6
Cauldren Foods Organic or Original Tofu, one-third of 250g pack	4	6
Egg, 1 medium	3	6
Frankfurter/Hot Dog, e.g. Tivall, Sainsbury, Tesco	3	5
Meat Free Burger, frozen, average	3.5	3
Pulses, canned, average for all types, 1 rounded tbsp	1	0
Quorn Bacon Style Rasher, each	1	1
Quorn Burger, frozen, each	3	2.5
Quorn Deli Slices, all flavours, 2 slices	1	0.5
Quorn Lamb Style Grill, chilled, each	4	3
Quorn Mince or Pieces, raw, 100g	4	2.5
Quorn Peppered Steak, chilled, each	4	4
Quorn Sausage, frozen, each	2	2
Tivall Vegetarian Mince, 100g	6	6

Cheese, Soft	Checks	Fat g
Cheese Spread Triangle, half-fat, 14-17g	1	1.5
Cottage Cheese, 25g	1	1
Cottage Cheese, half-fat, 25g	1	0.5
Curd Cheese, 25g	2	3
Philadelphia Extra Light Mini, 35g pot	1.5	2
Processed Cheese Slice, half-fat, 20g	1.5	2
Quark Skimmed Milk Soft Cheese, 25g	1	0
Roulé, half-fat, 25g	2	3
Soft Cheese Extra Light, 25g	1	1.5
Soft Cheese Light, 25g	2	5

Cheese, Hard	Checks	Fat g
Babybel Mini Light, 1	2	2.5
Cheddar, 3% fat, 30g	2.5	1
Cheddar, half-fat, 30g	3	5
Edam, half-fat, 30g	3	3
Feta/Greek Style, half-fat, 30g	2	2.5
Leerdammer Lightlife, 28g slice	3	5
Mozzarella, half-fat, 30g	2.5	3
Président 9% fat Light Slices, 16.8g slice	1.5	1.5

Know what's low (cont'd)

Savoury Snacks	Checks	Fat g
Boots Shapers Crunchy Onion Rings, 12g bag	2.5	3.5
Boots Shapers Lightly Salted Potato Tubes, 15g bag	2.5	3
Boots Shapers Prawn Spirals, 19g bag	3	3
Breadstick (Grissini), 1	1	0.5
Carr's Table Water Biscuits, 2	1	0.5
Crackerbread, 2	1.5	0.5
Finn Crisp Multigrain Crispbread, 1	1	0.5
Jacob's Cream Cracker Light, 1	1	0.5
Melba Toasts, 20g pack of 6	3	0.5
Paterson's Oat Bites, 2	1	1
Paterson's Mixed Herb Oat Cracker, 1	1	1
Rice Cake, 1	1	0
Ryvita Dark Rye or Original Crispbread, 1	1	0
Sainsbury's BGTY Crispy Potato Bites, 20g bag	3	0.5
Sainsbury's BGTY Rosemary & Sea Salt Pita Chips, 20g bag	3	0.5
Snack-a-Jacks Jumbo Barbecue or Cheese, 1	1.5	0.5
Snack-a-Jacks Popcorn, Light Salted or Salt & Vinegar, 13g bag	2	1.5
Snapz Vegetable Crisps, 20g bag	3	0
Walkers Frazzles, 25g bag	3	4
Walkers French Fries, 19g bag	3	3

Sweet Treats	Checks	Fat g
Aero Milk Chocolate or Mint Mini, 11g	2	3
Alpen Light Cereal Bar, 1	2.5	1
Asda Good For You! Date & Walnut Cake Slice, 1	2.5	0.5
Cadbury's Light Chocolate Mousse, 55g pot	2.5	2
Carte d'Or Light Vanilla Ice Cream, 60ml scoop	1.5	1.5
Chupa Chups Cremosa Sugar-free Lolly, 1	1	0.5
Del Monte Fruitini Fruit Juice Lolly	2	0
Mackie's Iced Fruit Smoothie, 60ml tube	2	0.5
Marks & Spencer COU Chocolate Mousse, 70g pot	3	2
Marks & Spencer COU Lemon or Raspberry Mousse, 70g pot	3	2
Meringue Nest, 1	2	0
Mini Meringue, 1	0.5	0
Ready-to-eat Semi-dried Apricots or Prunes, 50g	3	0
Ryvita Goodness Cereal Bar (not Luxury), 1	2.5	0.5
Sainsbury's BGTY Apple Chips, 15g bag	2	0
Sainsbury's BGTY Cake Slices, all flavours, 1	2.5	0.5
Skinny Cow Strawberries & Cream Stick	3	1
Snack-a-Jacks Jumbo Delights, 1	2.5	1
Snapz Apple Crisps, 20g bag	3	0
Snapz Mini Snapz, 14g bag	2	0
Terry's Chocolate Orange, 1 segment	2	2.5
Tesco Light Choices Lemon Drizzle or Toffee Cake Slice, 1	3	0.5
Wall's Milk Time Mini Milk, 1	1	1

Then size 20

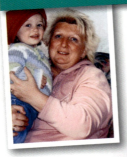

Sally Mitchell

" I set myself a secret target of wearing a size 14, red dress at my Ruby Wedding – and I did it! "

Weight loss:
5 stone 10½ lbs

Now size 14